CHAIR YOGA FOR SENIORS

Embrace Fitness, Flexibility, and Serenity at Any Age

Table of contents

Introduction to Chair Yoga

As we age, maintaining physical activity becomes increasingly important for overall health and well-being. However, traditional forms of exercise may feel intimidating or out of reach for those with limited mobility, chronic conditions, or balance issues. This is where chair yoga comes in—a gentle, accessible, and effective form of yoga that allows seniors to reap the physical and mental benefits of yoga while sitting comfortably on a chair. Let's explore what chair yoga is, why it's especially beneficial for seniors, and who can practice it.

What Is Chair Yoga?

Chair yoga is a modified form of yoga that is performed while seated in a chair or using a chair for support during standing poses. Unlike traditional yoga, which often involves movements on the floor or challenging balancing postures, chair yoga adapts classic yoga poses to make them safer and more accessible for people of all abilities.

In a typical chair yoga session, participants move through gentle stretches, twists, forward bends, and even standing poses while holding onto the chair for support. These movements are often paired with mindful breathing techniques and relaxation exercises to create a holistic practice that benefits both the body and mind.

Chair yoga retains the core principles of yoga—building strength, improving flexibility, and promoting mental clarity—without the physical demands of traditional yoga classes. This makes it an ideal form of exercise for seniors looking for a low-impact way to stay active.

Benefits of Chair Yoga for Seniors

Chair yoga offers a wide range of benefits that cater to the unique needs of seniors. These include:

1. Improved Flexibility and Mobility

Chair yoga gently stretches muscles and joints, helping to improve range of motion and reduce stiffness. This can make everyday activities like bending, reaching, or turning easier and more comfortable.

2. Increased Strength

Many chair yoga poses engage the core, legs, and arms, helping to build strength without putting excessive strain on the body. Stronger muscles can improve balance and reduce the risk of falls.

3. Enhanced Balance and Stability

Using a chair for support allows seniors to safely practice poses that improve balance. Over time, this can boost confidence in daily activities and decrease the likelihood of accidents.

4. Reduced Pain and Stiffness

Chair yoga is particularly beneficial for seniors dealing with conditions like arthritis, as it helps alleviate joint pain and inflammation through gentle, controlled movements.

5. Better Posture

Many chair yoga exercises focus on spinal alignment and core engagement, which can help counteract the effects of prolonged sitting or slouching.

6. Improved Circulation

The combination of movement and breathing in chair yoga promotes better blood flow, which is essential for heart health and overall vitality.

7. Stress Relief and Mental Clarity
Chair yoga incorporates mindfulness and breathing techniques that help reduce stress, anxiety, and depression. Regular practice can improve focus, memory, and overall mental well-being.

8. Accessible to All Fitness Levels
Whether you're an experienced yogi or completely new to yoga, chair yoga provides an entry point for everyone. Its adaptability ensures that no one is left behind.

Who Can Practice Chair Yoga?

One of the greatest strengths of chair yoga is its inclusivity. It is designed for individuals of all ages, abilities, and fitness levels. Seniors, in particular, can benefit from this practice, especially if they face the following challenges:

1. Limited Mobility

Seniors with mobility issues, whether due to aging, injury, or chronic conditions, can safely perform chair yoga without the need to get down on the floor.

2. Chronic Conditions

Chair yoga is ideal for those managing conditions like arthritis, osteoporosis, diabetes, or heart disease. It provides a gentle way to stay active without overexertion.

3. Balance Issues

Using a chair for support eliminates the fear of falling, allowing seniors to work on balance in a safe environment.

4. Recovering from Injury or Surgery

Chair yoga can be a great option for those recovering from surgery or an injury, as it allows them to stay active while minimizing strain on the body.

5. New to Yoga

Those who have never tried yoga before may find chair yoga to be a comfortable and approachable starting point.

6. Looking for Stress Relief

Chair yoga isn't just about physical health; it's also a powerful tool for calming the mind. Seniors seeking emotional balance or stress relief can find solace in the practice.

In essence, chair yoga is for anyone who wants to improve their physical and mental health in a gentle, supportive way. It's a practice that meets you where you are and encourages you to move at your own pace.

Chair yoga is more than just a workout; it's a gateway to a healthier, happier life. Whether you're looking to enhance your flexibility, build strength, or simply find a moment of peace in your day, chair yoga offers something for everyone. In the next sections, we'll dive deeper into specific poses, routines, and techniques that will help you make the most of this transformative practice.

Chapter 1: Getting Started with Chair Yoga

Embarking on a chair yoga journey is an exciting step toward better physical and mental well-being. But like any new activity, setting yourself up for success requires a little preparation. This section will guide you through selecting the right chair, understanding essential safety tips, and creating a comfortable practice space to make your chair yoga experience both enjoyable and effective.

Choosing the Right Chair

Your chair is the foundation of your practice, so choosing the right one is essential for comfort, stability, and safety. Here are the key factors to consider when selecting your chair:

1. **Stability**

- Opt for a sturdy chair with four legs and no wheels. Chairs with wheels or unstable bases can slide or tip over, increasing the risk of injury.

- Wooden or metal chairs often provide better stability than lightweight plastic ones.

2. Height

- The chair should allow you to sit with your feet flat on the floor and your knees bent at a 90-degree angle. This position ensures proper alignment and balance during poses.

- If the chair is too high, use a yoga block, cushion, or folded blanket under your feet for support.

3. Seat Surface

- Choose a chair with a flat, firm seat rather than a cushioned or slanted one. A firm surface provides better support for your posture and movements.

- Avoid chairs with armrests that can restrict your range of motion during poses.

4. Backrest

- If possible, select a chair with a straight backrest to support your spine during seated poses. Avoid chairs with overly reclined or curved backs.

5. Optional Features

- Chairs with non-slip rubber caps on the legs can prevent sliding, especially on smooth surfaces.

- If you have balance concerns, chairs with a slightly wider base may feel more secure.

By choosing the right chair, you'll ensure a safe and enjoyable foundation for your practice.

Safety Tips for Practicing Chair Yoga

Safety is a top priority when practicing chair yoga, especially for seniors or those with mobility challenges. Follow these tips to maximize your safety and confidence:

1. **Warm-Up First**

- Always start with a gentle warm-up to prepare your muscles and joints for movement. Simple shoulder rolls, neck stretches, or seated marches can help loosen up your body.

2. Listen to Your Body

- Pay attention to how your body feels during each pose. If a movement causes pain or discomfort, stop immediately and modify the pose as needed. Yoga should never hurt—it's about finding ease and comfort in your practice.

3. Practice Slow, Controlled Movements

- Avoid sudden or jerky movements that could strain your muscles or joints. Move slowly and mindfully to maintain balance and control.

4. Use Support When Needed

- If you're trying a standing pose, use the chair for support to avoid losing balance. Holding onto the backrest or seat can provide stability and confidence.

5. Avoid Overstretching

- It's tempting to push yourself, but overstretching can lead to injury. Move only as far as your body comfortably allows and gradually build flexibility over time.

6. Wear Comfortable Clothing

- Choose loose, breathable clothing that allows for a full range of motion. Avoid tight waistbands or garments that restrict movement.

7. Stay Hydrated

- Keep a bottle of water nearby to stay hydrated, especially if you're practicing in a warm environment.

8. Practice in a Safe Environment

- Ensure your practice area is free of clutter, loose rugs, or other tripping hazards.

9. Consult a Professional

- If you have any medical conditions or concerns, consult your doctor before beginning chair yoga. A qualified yoga instructor can also guide you on proper alignment and modifications.

Setting Up Your Practice Space

Creating a comfortable and inviting practice space is essential for a focused and enjoyable chair yoga session. Here's how to design your space:

1. Choose a Quiet Area

- Select a quiet spot in your home where you won't be interrupted. This helps create a calming environment for mindfulness and relaxation.

2. Adequate Space

- Ensure there's enough space around your chair to move freely, especially for poses that involve extending your arms or legs. Aim for at least 3 feet of clearance in all directions.

3. **Non-Slip Flooring**

- Practice on a surface with good traction, like a yoga mat or non-slip rug. Avoid practicing on slippery floors, as this could cause the chair to slide.

4. **Good Lighting**

- Make sure the area is well-lit to help you see and follow your movements clearly. Natural light can enhance the calming atmosphere of your practice.

5. **Add Comforting Elements**

- Enhance the ambiance with items like soft lighting, candles, or calming music. A peaceful environment can make your practice more enjoyable.

6. Keep Props Handy

- Have yoga props such as blocks, straps, or cushions within reach. These can be helpful for modifying poses and providing extra support.

7. Set a Timer

- If you're practicing on your own, set a timer to manage your session. This helps you stay focused and ensures you dedicate enough time to each part of your routine.

8. **Personal Touches**

- Add items that bring you joy, such as plants, artwork, or a favorite quote. These personal touches can make your practice space feel welcoming and inspiring.

By selecting the right chair, prioritizing safety, and creating a comfortable practice space, you'll set yourself up for a successful and rewarding chair yoga journey. In the following sections, we'll explore specific poses and routines to help you get the most out of your practice.

Chapter 2: Breathing Techniques for Relaxation

Breathing is a natural and automatic process that sustains life, but how often do we stop to truly focus on the way we breathe? In chair yoga, breathing is much more than an unconscious action—it's a tool for relaxation, mental clarity, and emotional balance. Learning how to control and deepen your breath can transform not only your yoga practice but also your overall well-being.

In this section, we'll explore simple breathing exercises, the role of breath in yoga, and how it can serve as a powerful tool for stress relief.

Simple Breathing Exercises

Here are some beginner-friendly breathing techniques you can incorporate into your chair yoga practice:

1. Diaphragmatic Breathing (Belly Breathing)

- **What It Is**: A calming exercise that focuses on engaging your diaphragm for deep, restorative breaths.

- **How to Do It**:

  1. Sit upright in your chair with your feet flat on the floor. Place one hand on your chest and the other on your belly.

  2. Inhale deeply through your nose, allowing your belly to rise while keeping your chest still.

3. Exhale slowly through your mouth, feeling your belly fall.

4. Repeat for 5–10 breaths, focusing on the rhythm and depth of each inhale and exhale.

- **Benefits**: Reduces stress, promotes relaxation, and improves lung function.

2. Equal Breathing (Sama Vritti)

- **What It Is:** A balancing breath technique where the inhale and exhale are of equal length.

- **How to Do It:**

1. Sit comfortably and close your eyes if you're comfortable doing so.

2. Inhale slowly through your nose for a count of 4.

3. Exhale slowly through your nose for a count of 4.

4. Gradually extend the count to 5 or 6 as you become more comfortable.

5. Practice for 1–3 minutes.

- **Benefits**: Promotes focus, balances the nervous system, and reduces anxiety.

3. Alternate Nostril Breathing (Nadi Shodhana)

- **What It Is**: A cleansing breath that helps balance the body's energy channels.

- **How to Do It:**

1. Sit upright and use your right thumb to close your right nostril.

2. Inhale deeply through your left nostril.

3. Close your left nostril with your ring finger and release your thumb from the right nostril.

4. Exhale through your right nostril.

5. Inhale through your right nostril, close it, and exhale through the left nostril.

6. Repeat for 5–10 cycles.

- **Benefits**: Clears the mind, reduces stress, and restores balance.

4. Cooling Breath (Sitali)

- **What It Is:** A refreshing breath that helps cool the body and calm the mind.

- **How to Do It:**

1. Sit comfortably and curl your tongue into a tube (or purse your lips if you can't curl your tongue).

2. Inhale slowly through your tongue or pursed lips, feeling the cooling sensation.

3. Exhale slowly through your nose.

4. Repeat for 8–10 breaths.

- **Benefits**: Reduces stress, cools the body, and improves focus.

The Importance of Breath in Yoga

Breathing is the foundation of any yoga practice, including chair yoga. In yoga philosophy, the breath is referred to as "prana," meaning life force or vital energy. By controlling the breath, we can influence how energy flows through our body and mind.

1. Connection Between Breath and Movement

- In yoga, each movement is synchronized with the breath. For example, you may inhale to lengthen the spine and exhale to twist or fold. This coordination creates a sense of mindfulness and fluidity in your practice.

2. Enhances Mind-Body Awareness

- Focusing on the breath helps anchor your attention to the present moment, fostering a deeper connection between the mind and body.

3. Regulates the Nervous System

- Conscious breathing activates the parasympathetic nervous system, which is responsible for the body's "rest and digest" state. This helps lower heart rate, reduce blood pressure, and promote relaxation.

4. Supports Physical Poses

- Deep, controlled breathing provides stability and endurance during poses, allowing you to hold them longer and with greater ease.

Breath is the bridge that connects the physical and mental aspects of yoga. Mastering this connection can elevate your practice and improve your overall well-being.

Breathing for Stress Relief

Stress is an inevitable part of life, but how we respond to it can make all the difference. Breathing techniques are among the most effective tools for managing stress and cultivating a sense of calm.

1. **Activates the Relaxation Response**

   - Deep breathing signals the brain to shift from the "fight or flight" response to the "rest and digest" state, helping to calm both the mind and body.

2. **Reduces Muscle Tension**

   - Stress often causes physical tension, especially in the shoulders, neck, and jaw. Focused breathing helps release this tension, leaving you feeling more at ease.

3. Improves Emotional Regulation

- When you're feeling overwhelmed, slowing down your breath can help you pause, reflect, and respond to situations with greater clarity and composure.

4. Encourages Mindfulness

- Breathing exercises help bring your attention to the present moment, breaking the cycle of anxious or negative thoughts.

One simple practice for stress relief is the **4-7-8 Breathing Technique:**

- Inhale through your nose for a count of 4.

- Hold your breath for a count of 7.

- Exhale through your mouth for a count of 8.

- Repeat for 3–5 cycles to calm the mind and body.

By incorporating these breathing techniques into your chair yoga practice and daily routine, you can create a powerful toolset for relaxation and stress relief. In the next sections, we'll explore how to integrate these breathing exercises with yoga poses to enhance your physical and mental well-being.

Chapter 3: Foundational Poses

Chair yoga offers a gentle and accessible way to improve flexibility, strength, and balance while minimizing the risk of injury. Mastering foundational poses sets the stage for a safe and rewarding practice. This section introduces gentle warm-up stretches, key poses for beginners, and tips on achieving proper alignment while avoiding common mistakes.

Gentle Warm-Up Stretches

Before diving into chair yoga poses, it's essential to prepare your body with simple warm-up stretches. These movements help loosen tight muscles, improve circulation, and reduce stiffness, especially for seniors.

1. **Neck Rolls**

- **How to Do It:**

1. Sit upright with your feet flat on the floor and hands resting on your thighs.

2. Gently drop your chin toward your chest.

3. Slowly roll your head to the right, bringing your ear toward your shoulder.

4. Roll your head back to the center, then to the left.

5. Repeat 3–5 times in each direction.

- **Benefits**: Relieves neck tension and increases flexibility.

2. Shoulder Rolls

- **How to Do It:**

  1. Sit upright with your arms at your sides.

  2. Inhale and lift your shoulders toward your ears.

  3. Exhale as you roll your shoulders back and down.

  4. Repeat 5 times, then reverse the direction.

- **Benefits**: Loosens tight shoulders and improves posture.

3. Seated Cat-Cow Stretch

- **How to Do It**:

  1. Sit with your feet flat on the floor and hands on your knees.

  2. Inhale, arch your back, and lift your chest and chin (Cow Pose).

  3. Exhale, round your spine, and tuck your chin toward your chest (Cat Pose).

  4. Repeat for 5–8 breaths.

- **Benefits**: Improves spinal flexibility and relieves back tension.

4. Seated Side Stretch

- **How to Do It:**

  1. Sit upright and place your right hand on the side of your chair.

  2. Inhale, raise your left arm overhead, and stretch to the right.

  3. Hold for a few breaths, then return to center and switch sides.

- **Benefits**: Stretches the sides of your torso and improves lateral flexibility.

5. Ankle Circles

- **How to Do It:**

  1. Sit with your feet flat on the floor.

  2. Lift one foot slightly off the ground and rotate your ankle in a circular motion.

  3. Do 5–10 circles in each direction, then switch to the other foot.

- **Benefits**: Enhances ankle mobility and promotes circulation.

Key Chair Yoga Poses for Beginners

Once your body is warmed up, you can move into foundational chair yoga poses. These beginner-friendly poses are designed to improve strength, flexibility, and balance while using the chair for support.

1. Seated Mountain Pose (Tadasana)

- **How to Do It:**

    1. Sit upright with your feet flat on the floor and hands resting on your thighs.

    2. Engage your core and lengthen your spine.

3. Relax your shoulders and lift the crown of your head toward the ceiling.

4. Breathe deeply and hold for 5–8 breaths.

- **Benefits**: Improves posture, focus, and body awareness.

2. Seated Forward Fold (Uttanasana)

- **How to Do It:**

1. Sit at the edge of your chair with your feet hip-width apart.

2. Inhale, then exhale as you hinge at your hips and fold forward,

letting your hands reach toward the floor.

3. Hold for a few breaths, then slowly rise back up.

- **Benefits**: Stretches the back, hamstrings, and shoulders.

3. Seated Spinal Twist (Ardha Matsyendrasana)

- **How to Do It:**

1. Sit upright with your feet flat on the floor.

2. Place your right hand on the backrest of the chair and your left hand on your right thigh.

3. Inhale, lengthen your spine, and exhale as you twist to the right.

4. Hold for a few breaths, then return to center and switch sides.

- **Benefits**: Enhances spinal flexibility and aids digestion.

4. Chair Warrior Pose (Virabhadrasana)

- **How to Do It:**

1. Sit sideways on the chair with your right leg bent and your left leg extended behind you.

2. Raise your arms overhead or extend them to the sides.

3. Hold for a few breaths, then switch sides.

- **Benefits**: Strengthens legs, improves balance, and opens the hips.

5. Seated Sun Salutation (Modified Surya Namaskar)

- **How to Do It:**

1. Start in Seated Mountain Pose.

2. Inhale, raise your arms overhead (Upward Salute).

3. Exhale, fold forward (Seated Forward Fold).

4. Inhale, place your hands on your thighs and lift your chest (Seated Cow Pose).

5. Exhale, round your spine (Seated Cat Pose).

6. Repeat for 3–5 cycles.

- **Benefits**: Increases energy and flexibility.

Proper Alignment and Common Mistakes

Correct alignment ensures you get the most out of each pose while minimizing the risk of injury. Here are some tips for

proper alignment and avoiding common
mistakes:

1. Posture

- **Do**: Sit upright with your spine long and shoulders relaxed.

- **Don't**: Slouch or lean too far forward or backward.

2. Breath Awareness

- **Do**: Coordinate your breath with your movements. Inhale during lengthening movements and exhale during folds or twists.

- **Don't**: Hold your breath during poses—it can cause tension and reduce the benefits.

3. Joint Safety

- **Do**: Keep your knees aligned with your ankles and avoid locking them.

- **Don't**: Overextend your joints or push through discomfort.

4. Core Engagement

- **Do**: Engage your core muscles to support your movements.

- **Don't**: Rely solely on your arms or legs for strength—use your whole body.

5. Modifications

- **Do**: Use props like cushions or yoga blocks for extra support.

- **Don't**: Force yourself into poses beyond your current flexibility or strength level.

By mastering these foundational poses, you'll build confidence, strength, and flexibility in your chair yoga practice. In the next section, we'll explore more advanced movements to deepen your experience while continuing to honor your body's needs.

Chapter 4: Chair Yoga Routines

Developing a consistent chair yoga practice can profoundly benefit your physical and mental well-being. This section outlines three practical and adaptable routines that cater to different time commitments and goals: a 10-minute energy boost for your mornings, a 20-minute routine to stretch and strengthen your body, and a 30-minute flow designed to relax your mind and enhance flexibility. These routines are suitable for seniors at any fitness level, with modifications provided to ensure accessibility.

10-Minute Morning Energy Boost

Kickstart your day with a quick chair yoga sequence that energizes your body, awakens your mind, and prepares you for the day ahead. This routine incorporates gentle stretches, mindful breathing, and dynamic movements to invigorate your system.

1. Seated Mountain Pose (1 Minute)

- Sit upright with your feet flat on the floor and your hands resting on your thighs.

- Lengthen your spine, relax your shoulders, and breathe deeply.

- Visualize energy flowing through your body with each inhale.

2. Seated Side Stretch (1 Minute)

- Place your right hand on the side of the chair and lift your left arm overhead.

- Stretch to the right, feeling the lengthening along your side.

- Hold for a few breaths, then switch sides.

3. Seated Cat-Cow (2 Minutes)

- Place your hands on your knees. Inhale, arch your back, and lift your chest (Cow Pose).

- Exhale, round your spine, and tuck your chin toward your chest (Cat Pose).

- Flow between these movements for 5–8 breaths.

4. Seated Spinal Twist (2 Minutes)

- Place your left hand on your right thigh and your right hand on the backrest of the chair.

- Inhale, lengthen your spine, and exhale as you twist to the right.

- Hold for a few breaths, then switch sides.

5. Seated Sun Salutation (4 Minutes)

- Start in Seated Mountain Pose.

- Inhale, raise your arms overhead.

- Exhale, fold forward toward your thighs.

- Inhale, rise back to an upright position.

- Repeat for 3–5 cycles, coordinating your breath with the movements.

20-Minute Stretch and Strengthen Routine

This intermediate routine combines stretching and strengthening exercises to enhance mobility, improve posture, and build muscle tone. It's ideal for mid-morning or afternoon sessions.

1. Neck Rolls (1 Minute)

- Gently roll your head in circular motions, first clockwise, then counterclockwise.

- Release any neck tension before moving on.

2. Shoulder Rolls (2 Minutes)

- Roll your shoulders forward and backward in slow, deliberate motions.

- This improves shoulder mobility and posture.

3. Seated Warrior I (3 Minutes)

- Sit sideways on the chair with your left leg bent and your right leg extended behind you.

- Raise your arms overhead and hold for several breaths.

- Repeat on the opposite side.

4. Seated Warrior II (3 Minutes)

- Remain in the same position as Warrior I but extend your arms to the sides at shoulder height.

- Gaze over your front hand and hold for several breaths on each side.

5. **Seated Forward Fold with Shoulder Stretch (4 Minutes)**

- Fold forward from your hips, letting your arms dangle toward the floor.

- Option: Interlace your fingers behind your back and lift your hands for a gentle shoulder stretch.

6. **Seated Leg Lifts (3 Minutes)**

- Sit upright and extend one leg straight out.

- Hold for a few breaths, then lower it.

- Repeat 5–8 times on each leg to strengthen your thighs and core.

7. Seated Side Bend with a Twist (4 Minutes)

- Combine a side stretch with a twist to enhance flexibility in your spine and core.

- Stretch your left arm overhead, twist slightly to the right, and hold.

- Switch sides and repeat.

30-Minute Relaxation and Flexibility Flow

This extended routine is perfect for evenings or whenever you want to unwind. It combines soothing poses and deep stretches to relax your mind and improve flexibility.

1. **Centering Breathwork (3 Minutes)**

- Sit comfortably and close your eyes.

- Take slow, deep breaths, focusing on your inhale and exhale.

- Let go of any tension or stress.

2. **Seated Eagle Arms (3 Minutes)**

- Wrap your right arm under your left and bring your palms together.

- Lift your elbows slightly and hold for a few breaths.

- Switch sides to stretch your shoulders and upper back.

3. **Seated Half Moon Pose (3 Minutes)**

- Lift your left arm overhead and stretch to the right.

- Hold for a few breaths, then switch sides.

- Focus on creating length through your side body.

4. **Seated Pigeon Pose (5 Minutes)**

- Place your right ankle on your left knee, forming a figure-four shape.

- Flex your foot and lean forward slightly for a deeper stretch.

- Hold for a minute, then switch sides.

5. Seated Forward Fold (5 Minutes)

- Hinge at your hips and fold forward, letting your arms dangle or rest on your legs.

- Take deep breaths and relax into the pose.

6. Seated Spinal Twist (5 Minutes)

- Perform a gentle twist to each side, holding for 1–2 minutes per side.

- Focus on your breath as you deepen the twist.

7. Seated Restorative Pose (6 Minutes)

- Sit upright with your hands resting on your thighs or in your lap.

- Close your eyes and take slow, deep breaths.

- Focus on relaxation and gratitude for your practice.

These chair yoga routines are designed to be flexible and adaptable to your needs. Whether you're seeking a quick energy boost, a strengthening session, or a relaxing flow, these sequences offer something for everyone. By incorporating these routines into your daily life, you'll enjoy the physical and mental benefits of a consistent yoga practice tailored to your comfort and abilities.

Chapter 5: Adapting Chair Yoga for Specific Needs

Chair yoga is an inclusive and flexible practice that can be tailored to meet the diverse needs of seniors. Whether you are dealing with arthritis, limited mobility, or balance challenges, this adaptable form of yoga provides gentle and effective exercises to support your health and well-being. This chapter explores ways to modify chair yoga for specific needs, ensuring it remains accessible, safe, and beneficial for everyone.

Yoga for Arthritis and Joint Pain

Arthritis and joint pain are common challenges for seniors, often leading to stiffness, reduced mobility, and discomfort. Chair yoga offers gentle stretches and movements designed to ease pain, increase joint flexibility, and improve circulation.

Benefits for Arthritis:

- Reduces stiffness and improves range of motion.

- Enhances joint lubrication through gentle movement.

- Strengthens muscles to support weakened joints.

- Promotes relaxation to ease pain and reduce stress.

Recommended Chair Yoga Poses for Arthritis:

1. Finger and Wrist Stretches

- Sit upright and extend one arm forward, palm up.

- Gently pull back your fingers with the opposite hand for a mild stretch.

- Switch sides and repeat to relieve stiffness in the hands and wrists.

2. Seated Knee Lifts

- While seated, lift one knee toward your chest, supporting it with your hands if needed.

- Hold for a few breaths and lower gently.

- This helps strengthen the muscles around the knees while maintaining joint mobility.

3. Ankle Rotations

- Lift one foot slightly off the floor and rotate your ankle in slow, circular motions.

- Rotate clockwise, then counterclockwise.

- This exercise promotes blood flow and reduces stiffness in the ankles.

4. Seated Shoulder Rolls

- Roll your shoulders forward and backward in slow, controlled movements.

- This reduces tension and stiffness in the shoulders and upper back.

Tips for Practicing Chair Yoga with Arthritis:

- Perform movements slowly and avoid pushing into pain.

- Focus on your breath to promote relaxation and body awareness.

- Use props, such as cushions, for added comfort and support.

Improving Balance and Stability

Balance tends to decline with age, increasing the risk of falls. Chair yoga can help seniors improve stability by strengthening the core, enhancing coordination, and increasing body awareness. Even seated poses can contribute to better balance, and chair-assisted standing poses offer additional benefits.

Benefits for Balance:

- Builds core strength, which is crucial for stability.

- Improves proprioception (awareness of body position).

- Increases confidence in movement.

Chair Yoga Exercises to Enhance Balance:

1. Seated Mountain Pose with Core Activation

- Sit upright with your feet flat on the floor and hands resting on your thighs.

- Engage your abdominal muscles and lengthen your spine.

- Hold for a few breaths to build core strength.

2. Chair-Assisted Tree Pose

- Sit sideways on the chair with one hand holding the backrest for support.

- Place the sole of one foot against your opposite ankle or shin (not the knee).

- Focus on a point ahead and balance for a few breaths before switching sides.

3. Heel-to-Toe Walk (Chair-Assisted)

- Stand behind the chair and hold the backrest for stability.

- Slowly walk heel-to-toe, placing one foot directly in front of the other.

- Focus on steady, deliberate movements to improve coordination.

4. Seated Side Bends with Arm Lifts

- Sit upright and stretch one arm overhead while bending gently to the side.

- This movement strengthens the sides of the torso, which are key to maintaining balance.

Tips for Practicing Balance Exercises:

- Use the chair for stability until you feel confident.

- Focus on slow, controlled movements to build strength.

- Perform balancing poses near a wall or sturdy surface for safety.

Modifications for Limited Mobility

Limited mobility, whether due to injury, illness, or chronic conditions, can make traditional yoga poses challenging. Chair yoga provides a supportive framework, allowing individuals to move comfortably while reaping the benefits of yoga.

Benefits for Limited Mobility:

- Increases circulation and reduces stiffness, even with minimal movement.

- Builds strength and flexibility without strain.

- Encourages relaxation and mental well-being.

Modified Chair Yoga Poses for Limited Mobility:

1. Seated Cat-Cow Stretch

- Place your hands on your thighs.

- Inhale, arch your back slightly, and lift your chest (Cow Pose).

- Exhale, round your spine, and tuck your chin (Cat Pose).

- This gentle movement promotes spinal flexibility.

2. Seated Leg Stretch with Support

- Sit upright and extend one leg forward, keeping the other foot flat on the floor.

- Flex your foot and gently lean forward for a hamstring stretch.

- Hold for a few breaths, then switch legs.

3. Arm Circles

- Extend your arms to the sides and make small circular motions.

- Gradually increase the size of the circles.

- This improves shoulder mobility and upper body strength.

4. Seated Side Stretch with Support

- Rest one hand on the side of the chair for stability.

- Stretch your opposite arm overhead and lean gently to the side.

- Keep the movement slow and comfortable.

Tips for Practicing Chair Yoga with Limited Mobility:

- Adjust poses to suit your range of motion and comfort level.

- Use props like pillows or straps for additional support.

- Focus on breathing deeply to enhance relaxation and oxygenate the body.

Chair yoga is a highly adaptable practice that can be tailored to meet various needs, from arthritis relief to balance improvement and modifications for limited mobility. By focusing on gentle movements, proper alignment, and mindful breathing, seniors can experience the physical and mental benefits of yoga without strain or discomfort. These adaptations empower individuals to embrace yoga as a tool for maintaining health, independence, and quality of life, regardless of physical limitations.

Chapter 6: Incorporating Mindfulness

Mindfulness and yoga go hand in hand, forming a powerful combination for mental clarity, relaxation, and emotional well-being. Chair yoga offers the perfect opportunity to integrate mindfulness into your practice, transforming simple movements into deeply restorative experiences. By focusing on the present moment, connecting with your breath, and embracing positivity, mindfulness can enhance both the physical and mental benefits of yoga. This chapter explores how to incorporate mindfulness into your chair yoga sessions through focused awareness, guided relaxation, and uplifting affirmations.

Practicing Mindfulness During Yoga

Mindfulness involves being fully present and aware of your thoughts, feelings, and sensations without judgment. When incorporated into chair yoga, mindfulness can help deepen your connection to your body and create a more meditative practice.

How to Practice Mindfulness During Yoga:

1. **Focus on Your Breath**:

- Begin each session with a few minutes of deep breathing.

- Notice the rhythm of your inhale and exhale, letting it guide your movements.

2. **Stay Present**:

- Pay attention to the sensations in your body as you move through each pose.

- Observe any tension, release, or warmth without trying to change it.

3. **Move with Intention**:

- Perform each movement slowly and deliberately, avoiding rush or force.

- Visualize the purpose of each pose, whether it's to stretch, strengthen, or relax.

4. **Engage All Your Senses**:

- Notice the feel of the chair beneath you, the sound of your breath, or the light in the room.

- Engaging your senses grounds you in the present moment.

Benefits of Mindfulness in Chair Yoga:

- Reduces stress and anxiety by calming the mind.

- Enhances body awareness, promoting better alignment and movement.

- Improves concentration and focus during practice and daily life.

Guided Relaxation Techniques

Guided relaxation, also known as yoga nidra or deep relaxation, is a meditative practice that fosters complete physical and mental rest. It can be done at the end of your chair yoga session to enhance relaxation and rejuvenation.

Steps for a Guided Relaxation Practice:

1. **Prepare Your Space:**

   - Sit comfortably in your chair, feet flat on the floor, and hands resting on your lap.

   - Close your eyes or soften your gaze.

2. **Body Scan Relaxation:**

   - Bring your attention to your head, noticing any tension in your forehead, jaw, or neck.

   - Gradually move your focus down through your shoulders, arms,

torso, legs, and feet, releasing
tension as you go.

3. Visualization for Relaxation:

- Imagine a peaceful scene, such as a calm beach, a forest, or a quiet garden.

- Picture yourself in this setting, noticing the sights, sounds, and sensations.

4. Breathing into Relaxation:

- Inhale deeply, imagining a wave of relaxation flowing through your body.

- Exhale, letting go of any lingering tension or worry.

5. Gratitude Practice:

- Conclude your relaxation by focusing on something you're grateful for, whether it's your health, loved ones, or the present moment.

Benefits of Guided Relaxation:

- Promotes deep relaxation and reduces stress.

- Enhances sleep quality and overall mental well-being.

- Provides a gentle transition from yoga practice to daily activities.

Affirmations for Positivity

Affirmations are positive statements that can shift your mindset, build self-confidence, and inspire joy.

Incorporating affirmations into your chair yoga practice can help you cultivate a positive outlook and strengthen your emotional resilience.

How to Use Affirmations During Yoga:

1. Start or End Your Session with Affirmations:

- Begin your practice by repeating a positive affirmation, such as, "I am strong and capable."

- Conclude your session by affirming gratitude or peace, such as, "I am grateful for this time for myself."

2. Pair Affirmations with Breathwork:

- As you inhale, silently say, "I am calm."

- As you exhale, say, "I let go of stress."

3. Integrate Affirmations with Movements:

- While lifting your arms overhead, think, "I welcome new energy."

- While folding forward, think, "I release what no longer serves me."

Examples of Positive Affirmations:

- "I honor my body and its unique journey."

- "I am present and at peace in this moment."

- "I trust my body's ability to heal and thrive."

- "I am strong, resilient, and full of vitality."

Benefits of Affirmations in Chair Yoga:

- Encourages a positive mindset and emotional balance.

- Strengthens the mind-body connection.

- Helps you set an intention for your practice and carry it into your day.

Incorporating mindfulness into your chair yoga practice transforms it into more than just physical movement—it becomes a holistic experience for your mind, body, and spirit. By staying present, practicing guided relaxation, and using affirmations, you can enhance the benefits of yoga while cultivating a deep sense of peace and positivity. This mindful approach empowers you to embrace each session with gratitude, joy, and self-compassion, enriching your overall well-being.

Chapter 7: Benefits of Each Pose

Chair yoga offers a wealth of benefits for both the body and mind, making it an ideal practice for seniors seeking to stay active, healthy, and balanced. Each pose in chair yoga is designed to address specific physical and mental needs while contributing to overall wellness. This chapter explores the physical, mental, and long-term benefits of chair yoga, focusing on how it supports healthy aging.

Physical Benefits: Strength, Flexibility, and Posture

Chair yoga poses are gentle yet effective exercises that strengthen muscles, enhance flexibility, and improve posture. These benefits are crucial for maintaining mobility and independence as we age.

1. Building Strength

- **How Chair Yoga Helps**: Many poses engage key muscle groups, including the legs, arms, core, and back, helping to maintain muscle tone and support joints.

- **Examples**:

  - **Seated Leg Lifts**: Strengthen the quadriceps and hip flexors, essential for walking and standing.

  - **Chair Push-Ups:** Build upper body strength, aiding in daily activities like lifting objects.

- **Why It's Important**: Strengthening muscles reduces the risk of falls and supports joint health, especially for those with arthritis or osteoporosis.

2. Increasing Flexibility

- **How Chair Yoga Helps**: Gentle stretches improve the range of motion in joints, making everyday movements smoother and easier.

- **Examples**:

  - **Seated Side Stretches**: Open up the sides of the torso, enhancing spinal flexibility.

  - **Seated Forward Fold:** Stretches the hamstrings and lower back, easing stiffness.

- **Why It's Important**: Improved flexibility prevents stiffness and reduces the likelihood of injuries.

3. Improving Posture

- **How Chair Yoga Helps**: Many poses focus on aligning the spine and strengthening the core, which are vital for good posture.

- **Examples**:

  - **Seated Mountain Pose**: Encourages an upright spine and engaged core.

  - **Seated Cat-Cow Stretch**: Promotes spinal mobility and awareness.

- **Why It's Important**: Proper posture minimizes back pain and enhances breathing, contributing to overall well-being.

Mental Benefits: Stress Reduction and Focus

Chair yoga isn't just about physical movement; it also nurtures the mind. Regular practice can significantly reduce stress, boost mood, and improve mental clarity.

1. Stress Reduction

- **How Chair Yoga Helps**: The combination of gentle movements and mindful breathing activates the parasympathetic nervous system, reducing stress and promoting relaxation.

- **Examples**:

- Seated Shoulder Rolls: Release tension in the shoulders and neck, common stress areas.

  - Breathing Techniques: Encourage calmness and mental clarity.

- **Why It's Important**: Chronic stress negatively impacts physical and mental health, making relaxation practices essential for overall wellness.

2. Enhancing Focus

- **How Chair Yoga Helps**: Mindful movement requires attention to the present moment, improving concentration and mental sharpness.

- **Examples**:

  - Balancing Poses (e.g., Chair-Assisted Tree Pose): Focus on stability and awareness.

  - Guided Relaxation: Centers the mind and increases awareness.

- **Why It's Important**: Enhanced focus and concentration improve problem-solving skills and memory, supporting cognitive health as we age.

3. Emotional Well-Being

- **How Chair Yoga Helps**: The practice fosters self-compassion and gratitude, contributing to emotional resilience and positivity.

Examples:

- ○ Affirmations During Yoga: Build a sense of self-worth and optimism.

- ○ Seated Heart Openers: Encourage openness and emotional release.

- **Why It's Important:** Emotional stability reduces the risk of anxiety and depression, common challenges for seniors.

How Yoga Supports Healthy Aging

Chair yoga is more than an exercise—it's a holistic approach to aging gracefully. It integrates physical activity, mental focus, and emotional well-being to support a vibrant, fulfilling life.

1. Promoting Longevity

- **How It Helps**: Regular physical activity like chair yoga improves cardiovascular health, lowers blood pressure, and enhances overall vitality.

- **Examples**:

    o Seated Spinal Twists: Support digestive health and spinal flexibility.

    o Ankle Rotations: Improve circulation and reduce swelling in the lower extremities.

- **Why It's Important**: Active seniors are more likely to enjoy a longer, healthier life.

2. Maintaining Independence

- **How It Helps**: Chair yoga strengthens the body and enhances coordination, making everyday tasks easier and safer.

- **Examples**:

    - Seated Core Twists: Build strength for bending and reaching.

    - Chair-Assisted Standing Poses: Improve balance for walking and standing.

- **Why It's Important:** Maintaining mobility and balance reduces the risk of falls, which are a major concern for aging individuals.

3. Encouraging Social Connection

- **How It Helps**: Chair yoga classes provide opportunities for community and social interaction, fostering a sense of belonging.

- **Examples**:

  - Group sessions encourage sharing experiences and mutual support.

- **Why It's Important**: Staying socially connected is vital for emotional health and cognitive function.

4. Enhancing Quality of Life

- **How It Helps**: The holistic benefits of chair yoga—physical strength, mental clarity, and emotional resilience—improve overall quality of life.

- **Examples**:

  - Morning Routines: Energize the body and mind for the day ahead.

  - Evening Relaxation Flows: Prepare for restful, restorative sleep.

- **Why It's Important**: Seniors who feel strong, focused, and content are better equipped to embrace the joys of aging.

Chair yoga offers transformative benefits for seniors, addressing both physical and mental health. From building strength and flexibility to reducing stress and supporting cognitive health, each pose is a step toward a healthier, more fulfilling life. By integrating chair yoga into your routine, you're not just practicing yoga—you're investing in your longevity, independence, and overall well-being. Healthy aging begins with small, intentional movements, and chair yoga provides the perfect foundation for a life well-lived.

Chapter 8: Real-Life Inspiration

Incorporating chair yoga into daily life can lead to remarkable transformations, not just physically but also mentally and emotionally. The beauty of chair yoga lies in its adaptability, making it accessible to people of all abilities and fitness levels. This chapter shines a light on real-life success stories from seniors who've embraced chair yoga and experienced its profound benefits. Their testimonials serve as an inspiration, showing that it's never too late to embark on a journey toward improved health and well-being.

Success Stories from Seniors Who Practice Chair Yoga

1. **Mary's Story: Rediscovering Mobility at 72**

Mary, a 72-year-old retired teacher, had struggled with arthritis for years. Simple tasks like bending to tie her shoes or reaching for items on a shelf became challenging. After joining a chair yoga class at her local senior center, Mary found a new sense of hope.

- **The Transformation**:

  - Within weeks, Mary noticed increased flexibility and reduced joint pain.

  - Poses like Seated Cat-Cow and Seated Forward Fold improved her spine's mobility.

- **Her Words:**

- "Chair yoga gave me my independence back. I can move without pain, and I even started gardening again!"

2. John's Story: Building Strength After Surgery

John, 68, underwent knee replacement surgery and was hesitant to return to physical activity. His physical therapist recommended chair yoga as a gentle way to regain strength.

- **The Transformation**:

  - Chair yoga poses such as Seated Leg Lifts and Chair-Assisted Warrior Pose helped him rebuild muscle strength and confidence.

- Breathing exercises calmed his anxiety about movement-related pain.

- **His Words**:

  - "I was skeptical at first, but chair yoga has been a game-changer. It's safe, effective, and has helped me feel strong again."

3. Anita's Story: Overcoming Isolation Through Yoga

At 76, Anita found herself feeling lonely after her children moved out of state. She joined a chair yoga class at a community center, hoping to meet new people and stay active.

- **The Transformation**:

- Yoga helped Anita manage stress and loneliness through mindfulness and relaxation techniques.

- Group classes provided her with a supportive social circle.

- **Her Words:**

  - "I not only improved my health, but I also made wonderful friends. Chair yoga gave me a community and a reason to smile."

4. Robert's Story: Managing Diabetes with Chair Yoga

Robert, a 70-year-old retired engineer, was diagnosed with type 2 diabetes. His doctor recommended regular physical activity to help manage his condition.

Chair yoga became a part of his daily routine.

- **The Transformation**:

  - Gentle movements like Seated Side Stretches and Chair-Assisted Sun Salutations helped improve his circulation and energy levels.

  - Deep breathing exercises reduced his stress, contributing to better blood sugar control.

- **His Words**:

  - "Chair yoga keeps my blood sugar stable and my mind at ease. It's the best decision I've made for my health."

Testimonials: How Yoga Transformed Their Lives

Susan, 65:
"Chair yoga has taught me to listen to my body and respect its limits. I used to think yoga was only for the young and flexible, but now I know it's for everyone. My balance has improved, and I feel more connected to myself."

Eleanor, 78:
"I've been doing chair yoga for two years, and it's become my favorite part of the day. The breathing exercises have helped me manage my anxiety, and the stretches have relieved my chronic back pain. I recommend it to all my friends!"

David, 69:
"After suffering from a stroke, I thought I'd never regain full mobility. Chair yoga helped me rebuild my strength and coordination. It's slow, steady, and

incredibly effective. I feel hopeful for the first time in years."

Barbara, 74:
"As a caregiver for my husband, stress was taking a toll on my health. Chair yoga gave me a way to care for myself while caring for him. It's my oasis of calm on a busy day."

Why These Stories Matter

These real-life accounts highlight the power of chair yoga to transform lives, proving that it's more than just an exercise—it's a pathway to physical recovery, mental clarity, and emotional resilience. These stories illustrate:

- The accessibility of chair yoga, no matter your age or physical condition.

- Its ability to address a wide range of challenges, from arthritis and diabetes to loneliness and stress.

- The supportive communities that chair yoga can foster, offering both health benefits and social connection.

The stories and testimonials in this chapter are a testament to the life-changing potential of chair yoga. Whether it's recovering from surgery, managing chronic conditions, or finding a sense of belonging, chair yoga offers something for everyone. These experiences remind us that small, consistent steps can lead to profound improvements in our overall well-being. Let these stories inspire you to start or continue your own journey with chair yoga—because it's never too late to transform your life.

Chapter 9: Taking Your Practice Further

As you continue your journey with chair yoga, there are countless ways to deepen your practice, enhance its benefits, and keep it fresh and exciting. In this chapter, we explore how adding props, building a consistent routine, and tapping into additional resources can take your chair yoga practice to the next level, helping you sustain progress and continue to reap the physical, mental, and emotional rewards of yoga.

Adding Props: Cushions, Resistance Bands, and More

Props are powerful tools that can support your chair yoga practice by providing extra stability, enhancing stretches, and helping you safely reach new levels of flexibility and strength.

Incorporating props into your routine can make certain poses more accessible, deepen your practice, and keep it engaging.

1. Cushions and Blocks

- **How They Help**: Cushions or yoga blocks provide support and alignment during seated poses, especially for those with limited flexibility or mobility. They can be placed under the hips, knees, or back to provide extra comfort and assist with maintaining proper posture.

- **Examples of Use:**

  - Place a cushion under your hips to elevate your seat in Seated Mountain Pose to ensure a neutral spine.

- o Use a cushion or block under the knees in seated stretches to prevent overstretching and relieve pressure on the joints.

- **Why It's Important**: Cushions help enhance comfort, making poses more accessible, and offer added support during long practice sessions.

2. Resistance Bands

- **How They Help**: Resistance bands are versatile tools that can strengthen muscles, improve flexibility, and increase the intensity of your yoga practice. They can be used to engage specific muscle groups, adding an extra challenge to your poses without needing weights.

- **Examples of Use:**

  - Loop a resistance band around your thighs for added resistance during seated leg lifts or Chair-Assisted Warrior Pose.

  - Use the band to gently deepen stretches, such as Seated Hamstring Stretch, by holding the band with your hands and gently pulling on your foot to deepen the stretch.

- **Why It's Important**: Resistance bands are ideal for building strength and flexibility in a controlled and safe way, making them a great tool for seniors who want to challenge themselves without straining their bodies.

3. Yoga Straps

- **How They Help**: Yoga straps are excellent for improving flexibility, especially in the legs and arms. They assist in reaching the feet or extending arms during stretches, helping to lengthen the muscles safely.

Examples of Use:

- Use a strap to hold your foot in the Seated Forward Fold if you're unable to reach your toes, allowing you to lengthen your hamstrings without strain.

- Loop a strap around your wrists during seated stretches to encourage proper arm alignment.

- **Why It's Important**: Yoga straps make it easier to deepen stretches and maintain proper form, which is crucial for avoiding injuries.

4. Chairs with Adjustable Features

- **How They Help**: A chair with adjustable height or armrests can help you find the perfect alignment for various poses. It can also offer additional stability for standing or balancing poses.

- **Examples of Use:**

  - Choose a chair with adjustable arms to allow for more space during seated twists or shoulder stretches.

- ○ Adjust the height to ensure your feet are flat on the floor in seated poses to promote proper posture.

- **Why It's Important**: A well-chosen chair can enhance comfort, stability, and the overall quality of your practice.

Building a Consistent Routine

Consistency is key when it comes to seeing progress in any yoga practice, and chair yoga is no different. Establishing a regular routine ensures that you continuously improve strength, flexibility, and mindfulness while creating a habit that integrates seamlessly into your life.

1. Setting Realistic Goals

- **How It Helps**: Having clear, achievable goals allows you to track progress and stay motivated. Goals can be as simple as practicing for a certain amount of time each day or mastering a specific pose.

- **Examples of Goals:**

  - Practice chair yoga for 10 minutes each morning to start your day with energy and focus.

  - Improve flexibility by gradually working on reaching further in seated stretches.

- **Why It's Important**: Setting goals gives you something to strive for and helps you stay focused, ensuring that your practice remains effective and fulfilling.

2. Establishing a Routine

- **How It Helps**: A set schedule makes it easier to incorporate chair yoga into your daily life. Try to practice at the same time each day, even if it's just for 10–15 minutes.

- **Tips for Consistency**:

  - Set a reminder on your phone or mark it in your calendar.

  - Choose a time that works best for you—morning, afternoon, or evening—when you feel most energized and focused.

- Keep your practice space inviting and accessible, so it's easy to practice regularly.

- **Why It's Important**: Consistency builds momentum and creates a lasting habit. Over time, you'll notice improvements in both your physical and mental well-being.

3. Varying Your Routine

- **How It Helps**: While consistency is key, it's also important to keep your practice fresh and engaging. Varying your routine helps you avoid stagnation and challenges different muscle groups.

- **Examples**:

- Alternate between different types of routines, such as a morning energy boost, a midday stretch, or an evening relaxation flow.

  - Experiment with adding props like resistance bands or cushions to keep poses dynamic.

- **Why It's Important**: Variety ensures that you engage your body in different ways, enhancing overall strength, flexibility, and balance.

Resources for Continued Learning

Yoga is a lifelong practice, and there's always more to learn. Fortunately, a wealth of resources is available to support you in expanding your knowledge, refining your practice, and exploring new techniques.

1. Online Yoga Classes and Tutorials

- **How They Help**: Many online platforms offer chair yoga classes for all levels, with clear instructions and guidance. You can join live sessions for a community experience or explore recorded videos to practice at your own pace.

- **Recommendations**:

  - Websites like Yoga with Adriene or Chair Yoga with Sherry offer great beginner-friendly sessions.

  - Check for free online courses or affordable subscriptions, such as those offered by local community centers or wellness platforms.

- **Why It's Important**: Online classes provide a structured way to continue learning while allowing flexibility to practice at home.

2. Yoga Books and Guides

- **How They Help**: Books provide in-depth explanations, photos, and tips on poses and techniques, making them an excellent resource for expanding your knowledge of chair yoga.

- **Recommendations**:

  - Look for books focused on chair yoga or yoga for seniors, such as Yoga for the Senior Body by Lynne B.

Minton or Chair Yoga: Sitting Yoga for Everyone by Kristi L. Reynolds.

- These resources offer step-by-step instructions and detailed descriptions to help deepen your practice.

- **Why It's Important**: Books provide a rich, thorough understanding of the philosophy behind yoga, which can enrich your physical practice.

3. Local Yoga Classes and Workshops

- **How They Help:** If possible, attending in-person classes or workshops can provide hands-on instruction and allow you to connect with other practitioners.

- **What to Look For:**

    - Look for chair yoga or senior yoga classes at local community centers, senior living facilities, or yoga studios.

    - Workshops or retreats can offer specialized, intensive learning experiences to enhance your practice.

- **Why It's Important**: Being part of a live class helps you receive feedback, ensures correct form, and fosters a sense of community.

4. Supportive Communities and Social Media

- **How They Help**: Engaging with other yoga practitioners online can provide inspiration, advice, and motivation. Join groups on social media or forums where you can share your experiences and learn from others.

- **Examples**:

  - Facebook groups or Instagram accounts dedicated to chair yoga for seniors.

  - Online forums where seniors share their yoga journeys and tips.

- **Why It's Important**: Community support encourages accountability and fosters a sense of belonging, which is essential for long-term success.

Taking your chair yoga practice further is about enhancing the depth and consistency of your routine, incorporating helpful props, and tapping into a wealth of resources to continue learning. With a commitment to regular practice, a willingness to explore new tools and techniques, and access to ongoing learning opportunities, you can deepen your practice and experience the full benefits of chair yoga. The more you invest in your practice, the more you'll discover how chair yoga can support your health, well-being, and overall quality of life. Keep growing, stay curious, and enjoy the journey!

Conclusion: Embracing Yoga for Life

Chair yoga is more than just a series of gentle stretches and movements. It's a practice that nurtures the body, calms the mind, and nurtures the soul, making it an invaluable tool for seniors seeking to live an active, healthy, and fulfilled life. As you reflect on your chair yoga journey and envision the path ahead, it's important to remember that yoga is not a destination—it's a lifelong practice that grows with you.

Reflecting on Your Chair Yoga Journey

Looking back on your time with chair yoga, you might be surprised by the transformations you've experienced—both big and small.

Perhaps you've noticed a newfound sense of flexibility, strength, or balance. Maybe you've experienced deeper relaxation, improved posture, or an enhanced sense of peace. These changes are the direct result of your commitment to moving your body and taking the time to nurture your well-being.

1. Celebrating Your Progress

Take a moment to celebrate how far you've come. Every pose you've mastered, every routine you've completed, and every new skill you've learned contributes to a healthier, happier you. It's easy to get caught up in what still needs to be achieved, but it's equally important to acknowledge the improvements you've made. Even if you haven't mastered every pose or routine, the consistency and effort you've put into your practice are what truly matter.

2. Embracing the Journey, Not the End Goal

Chair yoga is about much more than just physical results—it's about the journey itself. Yoga teaches us to embrace the present moment, to be mindful of our breath, and to be compassionate with ourselves. Every time you step onto your yoga mat (or into your chair), you're choosing to prioritize your health and happiness. In doing so, you're enriching your life in ways that go far beyond flexibility or strength. You're learning to embrace the process and enjoy the benefits that come with consistent practice, including emotional balance, mental clarity, and overall wellness.

3. Reflecting on the Mind-Body Connection

One of the most profound benefits of chair yoga is its ability to cultivate the mind-body connection. As you've learned through your practice, the body and mind are deeply intertwined. By paying attention to your breath, body movements, and emotions, you've probably noticed a reduction in stress and an improved sense of well-being. Chair yoga empowers you to be more in tune with yourself, and that awareness is a gift that will continue to enhance your life as you grow.

Staying Active, Healthy, and Happy

Chair yoga isn't just a practice—it's a way of life. It's a commitment to staying active, healthy, and happy as you age. Through your practice, you've already begun to reap the rewards of this mindful movement, and the journey doesn't end here. In fact, the more you integrate chair yoga into your daily routine, the more benefits you will experience, and the easier it will be to maintain a vibrant and joyful life.

1. The Lifelong Benefits of Staying Active

Physical activity is crucial for maintaining mobility, strength, and overall health as we age. Chair yoga provides a low-impact yet effective way to stay active and keep your body functioning at its best. As you continue practicing, you'll notice an increase in strength, flexibility, and balance—important factors in reducing the risk of falls and maintaining independence. The gentle nature of chair yoga means you can continue your practice at any stage of life, ensuring that you remain physically engaged and empowered, no matter your age or ability.

2. Prioritizing Mental and Emotional Well-Being

Yoga is not just for the body—it's for the mind and spirit, too. Chair yoga helps reduce anxiety, ease tension, and improve focus, leading to a clearer, calmer mind. As you continue to practice, remember that the benefits of mental clarity, emotional resilience, and stress reduction are just as important as the physical benefits. Staying emotionally balanced can improve your relationships, help you face challenges with grace, and contribute to an overall sense of happiness and fulfillment.

3. Finding Joy in Movement

One of the most beautiful aspects of chair yoga is its ability to transform even the simplest movements into opportunities for joy and self-care. Whether you're engaging in a morning routine, a midday stretch, or an evening relaxation flow, each practice offers a chance to reconnect with your body and mind. Embrace this sense of joy in movement, no matter how small or simple the action may seem. Even a few minutes of mindful stretching can have a profound impact on your mood, energy levels, and outlook on life.

E

The key to continuing your journey with chair yoga is making it a consistent part of your life. Whether you choose to practice daily, several times a week, or whenever you need a moment of calm, the important thing is to keep moving. Chair yoga offers flexibility in terms of time, space, and intensity, so you can tailor your practice to suit your unique needs and lifestyle. Create a routine that works for you, and stick with it. Over time, the more you practice, the easier it will be to integrate yoga into your daily habits and lifestyle.

5. Embracing the Holistic Benefits of Yoga

Yoga is a holistic practice that impacts not just the body but also the mind and spirit. By continuing to embrace chair yoga, you are investing in a full-spectrum approach to health and well-being. It's a practice that nurtures every aspect of you: physically, mentally, emotionally, and even spiritually. Chair yoga encourages you to slow down, listen to your body, and honor your own pace. As you move forward, remember that yoga is not just about achieving physical milestones; it's about finding peace, strength, and balance in every aspect of your life.

Looking Ahead: Your Ongoing Yoga Journey

As you conclude this chapter of your chair yoga journey, remember that it's only the beginning. Your practice will continue to evolve, and so will your ability to adapt it to your changing needs and goals. The key is to keep exploring, learning, and growing, both on and off the mat (or chair). With each practice, you'll deepen your connection to yourself and experience even greater benefits, physically, mentally, and emotionally.

Whether you are looking to maintain mobility, relieve stress, improve your posture, or simply find a moment of peace in your day, chair yoga is a valuable and life-affirming practice. Keep embracing the joy of yoga, stay mindful, and enjoy the journey toward a healthier, happier you.

Chair yoga is a powerful, accessible, and transformative practice that brings balance and well-being to all aspects of life. As you reflect on your journey and look ahead to the future, remember that yoga is about progress, not perfection. Stay committed, stay curious, and most importantly, stay present. Embrace yoga as a lifelong companion on your journey to health, happiness, and vitality.

Appendix

FAQ: Common Questions About Chair Yoga

1. What is chair yoga, and how is it different from regular yoga?

Chair yoga is a modified form of traditional yoga that is designed to be practiced while seated or with the aid of a chair for support. It's especially beneficial for seniors or anyone with limited mobility, as it allows individuals to practice yoga without needing to get on the floor. Unlike regular yoga, chair yoga is low-impact and adaptable, with the goal of improving flexibility, strength, and mental clarity while being mindful of one's physical limitations.

2. Is chair yoga suitable for beginners?

Absolutely! Chair yoga is ideal for beginners, especially for those new to yoga or who have specific physical concerns. It offers a gentle introduction to the practice, allowing individuals to build confidence and learn foundational movements in a safe and accessible manner. Chair yoga can also be easily modified for different levels of fitness, making it suitable for a wide range of abilities.

3. Can chair yoga help with back pain?

Yes, chair yoga can be highly beneficial for individuals dealing with back pain. The gentle stretches and movements involved in chair yoga help improve posture, strengthen the muscles around the spine, and increase flexibility, all of which can reduce discomfort and prevent further strain. However, it's important to listen to your body and avoid any movements that cause pain. Consulting with a healthcare provider before starting a new exercise routine is always a good idea.

4. How often should I practice chair yoga?

For best results, aim to practice chair yoga at least three to five times a week. Even practicing for just 10-15 minutes a day can have noticeable benefits. As you get more comfortable with the poses and movements, you may choose to increase the duration of your sessions or add more challenging exercises. Consistency is key to reaping the full benefits of yoga.

5. Can chair yoga help with stress and anxiety?

Yes, chair yoga is an excellent tool for managing stress and anxiety. Many of the techniques used in chair yoga, such as deep breathing and mindful movements, are proven to reduce stress and promote relaxation. Incorporating chair yoga into your daily routine can help calm the mind, enhance emotional well-being, and improve overall mental health.

6. Do I need any special equipment to practice chair yoga?

For basic chair yoga, all you really need is a sturdy chair. A yoga mat may be helpful for cushioning your feet or providing added support if you choose to stand for certain poses. You can also use props such as cushions, blankets, resistance bands, or yoga blocks to enhance comfort and support during your practice. These props can make certain poses easier and more accessible, especially if you have specific physical needs.

7. Is chair yoga safe for seniors?

Yes, chair yoga is safe for seniors, as it is specifically designed to be gentle and adaptable to various abilities. It offers a low-impact way to improve strength, balance, and flexibility without the risk of injury that may be associated with more intense forms of exercise. However, it's always advisable to consult with a healthcare provider before beginning any new exercise program, especially if you have underlying health concerns.

Additional Resources (Videos, Websites, and Apps)

For those who are eager to deepen their chair yoga practice, there are plenty of resources available to provide guidance and inspiration. Below are a selection of helpful videos, websites, and apps to support your journey:

1. Videos and YouTube Channels

- **Yoga With Adriene (Chair Yoga Playlist)**

Adriene Mishler's YouTube channel offers a variety of yoga tutorials, including a dedicated playlist for chair yoga. Adriene's clear instructions, soothing voice, and accessible approach make her videos perfect for beginners and seniors. You can follow along with her chair yoga sessions to improve your flexibility, strength, and relaxation.

- **Sit and Be Fit (YouTube Channel)**

Sit and Be Fit is a well-known program that offers chair-based exercises for seniors, including chair yoga. The videos focus on improving balance, flexibility, and strength while remaining easy to follow. This channel is great for individuals who are just getting started with yoga or those who prefer a slow and methodical approach.

- **Yoga Journal (Chair Yoga for Seniors Video Series)**

Yoga Journal's chair yoga video series is designed to help seniors enjoy the benefits of yoga with modifications for different abilities. With an emphasis on proper alignment and mindfulness, these videos guide you through a variety of poses that focus on strength, balance, and relaxation.

2. Websites

- **Yoga for Seniors (www.yogaforseniors.com)**

This website is a valuable resource for seniors who want to incorporate yoga into their daily lives. It offers tutorials, tips, and articles specifically for older adults, focusing on gentle poses that improve strength, flexibility, and mental clarity. Whether you're new to yoga or have experience, this site is an excellent starting point.

- **Chair Yoga with Peggy Cappy (www.peggy cappy.com)**

Peggy Cappy is a well-known chair yoga teacher who has created a series of online classes for seniors. Her website provides access to instructional videos, tips, and downloadable resources to help you practice chair yoga from the comfort of your home. The emphasis is on gentle movement, relaxation, and building strength.

- **SilverSneakers (www.silversneakers.com)**

SilverSneakers is a fitness program that offers chair yoga classes designed for older adults. Their website provides access to live classes, as well as a library of on-demand videos that focus on flexibility, strength, and mobility. It's an excellent platform for seniors who want to stay active and healthy.

3. Apps

- **Yoga for Beginners (App Store and Google Play)**

This app is designed for beginners and offers a variety of yoga routines, including chair yoga. It provides step-by-step instructions and illustrations to guide you through each pose. With customizable routines based on your fitness level, this app is a great option for those looking for a simple way to practice chair yoga on the go.

- **Down Dog (App Store and Google Play)**

Down Dog is a popular yoga app that offers various types of yoga, including chair yoga. The app features a wide range of difficulty levels and styles, allowing you to tailor your practice to your needs. It also offers a unique feature where you can choose the length of your session, making it easy to fit yoga into your busy schedule.

- **Daily Yoga (App Store and Google Play)**

Daily Yoga provides a comprehensive collection of yoga routines for all levels, including chair yoga options for seniors. It includes clear instructions, visual guides, and meditation practices to enhance your experience. You can also track your progress and receive reminders to practice regularly.

By using these resources, you can continue to expand your knowledge, refine your practice, and stay motivated as you explore the world of chair yoga. Whether you prefer watching instructional videos, following along with an app, or reading articles online, there's something for everyone to deepen their understanding and enjoy the many benefits of yoga for life.

Index

This Index provides a detailed reference to the essential topics covered in the book, guiding you quickly to the areas you wish to explore or revisit. Whether you're looking for specific poses, understanding the benefits of chair yoga, or finding answers to your questions, this index will help you navigate through the material efficiently.